The Weight Loss Diet Guide
Simple Strategies That Work

By: Patrick Withrow

Copyright 2015 by Washington Flamingo- All rights reserved.

This document is geared towards providing exact and reliable information in regards to the topic and issue covered. The publication is sold with the idea that the publisher is not required to render accounting, officially permitted, or otherwise, qualified services. If advice is necessary, legal or professional, a practiced individual in the profession should be ordered.

From a Declaration of Principles which was accepted and approved equally by a Committee of the American Bar Association and a Committee of Publishers and Associations.

In no way is it legal to reproduce, duplicate, or transmit any part of this document in either electronic means or in printed format. Recording of this publication is strictly prohibited and any storage of this document is not allowed unless with written permission from the publisher. All rights reserved.

The information provided herein is stated to be truthful and consistent, in that any liability, in terms of inattention or otherwise, by any usage or abuse of any policies, processes, or directions contained within is the solitary and utter responsibility of the recipient reader. Under no circumstances will any legal responsibility or blame be held against the publisher for any reparation, damages, or monetary loss due to the information herein, either directly or indirectly.

Respective authors own all copyrights not held by the publisher.

The information herein is offered for informational purposes solely, and is universal as so. The presentation of the information is without contract or any type of guarantee assurance.

The trademarks that are used are without any consent, and the publication of the trademark is without permission or backing by the trademark owner. All trademarks and brands within this book are for clarifying purposes only and are the owned by the owners themselves, not affiliated with this document.

Table of Contents

Introduction	1
Chapter One - **The First Steps**	5
Chapter Two - **Eliminate Stress**	17
Chapter Three - **Daily Goals, Systems and Routines**	21
Chapter Four - **Surround Yourself with the Greats**	27
Chapter Five- **Challenge Yourself**	31
Chapter Six- **Have a Vision, Collect Data and Progress**	33
Chapter Seven - **Importance of Exercise**	41
Chapter Eight - **Natural Supplements**	45
Conclusion	53
Join Our Facebook Groups	55

Introduction

Thank you for taking the time to read my book "The Weight Loss Diet Guide: Simple Strategies That Work". In this self-help weight loss book you are going to be provided with proven steps that have worked for me, but also my clients, friends and family. I have been passionate in the health and fitness industry for the last 10 years. I have spent many years personal training and working at supplement stores such as GNC and Complete Nutrition. A few years ago after being diagnosed with Crohn's disease I decided to make health and fitness my main priority in life because every day we have less time and if we are not improving our health on a day to day basis then we will not live as long. I have other priorities like my family, friends, businesses and a variety of hobbies, but every day I make sure I take time to be active so that I can hopefully have more time with the things that give me joy in my life. One of my main goals was to be able to write a book that is relatable and simple for people to follow and be able to achieve their health and fitness goals.

Everyone wants to feel loved; everyone wants to have a body they can show off, everybody wants to feel happy within them and to be able to accomplish this you will have to start with yourself. What do you want? Why do you want it? How will it make you feel? Embrace all the feelings and understand what you will have to do. What do you need to create in your life? What will you need to give up?

Burning fat is a difficult task. It's going to require you to spend a lot of time and a lot of effort on the process. If you have great intentions and you have the ability to really get to work you're going to be amazed at how quick and easy it is to see results. Take your time, take the initiative and know that you really can accomplish everything that you want for your life. You really can make yourself healthier and happier. You're the only one that can do it though. So take the initiative to start with this book, it's going to introduce you to everything you need and want in your life to create the body you envision for yourself.

Before you dive into this book I want you to take a few minutes to really think about what you want out of life. What body do you want? Why do you want this body? Who are you trying to impress? Why are you trying to impress them? When you achieve this sexy, gorgeous body what are you going to do with it? Are you going to the find the man or woman of your dreams? Are you going to play a professional sport, or get into modeling or compete in fitness competitions? Are you going to spend more time with your kids? What is the ultimate goal? Don't even stop at just your body. What is your lifestyle? How many days are you going to the gym? What kind of adventures are you seeking on the weekends? Are you hiking or horseback riding or doing sunrise yoga? Are you surrounding yourself with people that are athletic and eating healthy?

Don't stop at your health and fitness related dreams but are you financially free are you doing exactly what you want in life? Think of the ultimate goal that you want to achieve with your body and mind. Are you traveling? Are you hanging out with good mentors that are helping you create a more balanced life? Take these few minutes to really think about your end mind goal. What have you accomplished so far in life? What else would you like to accomplish? Write it down and get that visual of success to become crystal clear in your brain. Clarity is important and the more specific you can be towards a dream or goal the easier it will be to succeed. It is very important to do this because every single day you have one less chance of being who you want to be. It is never too late to start but if you never start you might live a long grueling life and you will wish you had done something.

Now I need you to stay in this state of mind and get ready to absorb this information. These strategies have helped me go from a frail skinny boy to the chiseled body I've always wanted. Then I took these steps into work and started helping my friends and family who were all shapes and sizes from being obese to sexy and from anorexic to strong and beautiful. If you're not in a good shape physically, don't get down because you're beautiful and not just in the inside. It's in all of you and if you haven't heard those words you need to start telling yourself that you are sexy, gorgeous, smart, funny, cool, bad ass or whatever makes you happy because starting out it will only be you but eventually people will see how determined you are. Chris Rock always said if his car broke down he would get out and push it because it would make people more inclined to help. God didn't breed us to be little bitches. He wants us to be great. He wants us to be proud of whom we are and he doesn't want us to leave anything on the table. Doesn't matter what God you believe in or what universe you believe in or ideas of life. At the end of the day this place wants us to be great. If you are reading this book it's because you are not satisfied with your life.

I believe in you. I've helped a lot of friends and clients achieve the body they wanted. It was never an overnight success, but it was the clients who stayed consistent. Understand that this is going to be the hardest thing ever to achieve and that everyone around you is going to get better and faster results, but if you stick with it then eventually you will you get there. You should already be happy though because life in itself is such a great gift. Embrace this journey, love the pain, love the results and show as much love towards yourself.

I love motivating people. I love coaching and training individuals to success. Success is different for each of us but if you can start today just by developing a crystal clear vision of the success that you want for your life then you are already progressing towards a better future. Use this book daily for whenever you need guidance. Being healthy and fit is not just for a month or three months. It has to be every day and you get to decide how to you want to be healthy and fit.

Just make sure you do it. Figure out your reasons and when it starts to get so fucking hard. I mean where you just want to fall on the ground and start crying because life decided not to be easy…Make sure you just keep going and keep moving forward. You will fail, you will fail a whole bunch but through those failures you are going to leave a legacy. A legacy that could be remembered by many or few, but regardless your life matters. Just make sure you do it.

Chapter One

The First Steps

When you start getting healthier and lose body fat the most important thing is to drink the amount of water your body needs. Your body is extremely sensitive and extremely intelligent as well. Unfortunately, it's not as intelligent as you might think. One way it's not as smart is that it isn't capable of differentiating between being hungry and needing water. As a result, you will be more inclined to eat something rather than drink water because your body treats the two the same way. You feel hungry when you don't even need food at all. I am definitely not saying to starve yourself, but if you do find that you are eating too much or eating too much of a certain type of food than my first step would be to try and get more water into your day to day life. I like drinking 32 ounces of water when I wake up and 32 ounces before I go to bed. I end up waking up in the middle of the night to pee, but it's worth it because I get to naturally detox my system from the horrible toxins that come into my body. You can also add a squeezed lemon into your water because when you drink it you actually alkaline the water into a healthier PH balance which will also help detox your body. I usually do regular water first and then sip on this because of its bitterness. Sounds weird because when you think of lemons you probably think of an acidic nature, but after I did much research from various sources it seems to work based off of the scientific studies that I looked at. I feel better mentally and physically as well. That could also be because how my state of mind is because of what I read or it could be because I am currently taking a break from alcohol until I hit a specific financial goal but all that I know is that it is a ritual that I have created for myself that I enjoy doing.

Remember it's about the rituals, systems and habits that you create for yourself that will make the biggest impact. The things that you do every single day will be what matter most. I started using my white board as a daily scheduler from 5 AM to 10 PM. I try my best to be a part of the 5 AM club on a consistent basis but every now and then when I am a DD for my friends on the weekends I will sometimes wake up a little bit later. It is all about balance as well. Don't try to be perfect, but remember consistency is the key to success in anything. The reason I do my best to wake up at 5 AM is because from 5 to 8 AM we have the most brain power. We are able to accomplish the most between the hours of 5 and 8 AM. If you look at most successful people they are usually up by 5 AM. What I did to motivate myself was writing down literally everything I did for every hour from 5 AM to 10 PM. When I realized the first couple days I was getting up at 9 AM or 10 AM I realized I missed all of this time. I would never be able to get back in my life again. It scared me because I never realized how precious my time was until I started writing down all of my production. Kirk Cousins breaks it down to every 15 minutes of his day and he color codes his daily scheduler which is awesome because I am a Redskins fan and that means we have a very hard working quarterback that is dedicating to bettering himself and the people he is around.

It may seem crazy to document everything and it might seem difficult, but it will help you develop better time management skills and I promise you if you manage your time better and write down all of your accomplishments it will become addicting to constantly succeed. It will become a game in your head where you will just constantly want to be better. I would highly recommend try using the white board or something to write down all of your habits, production, workout routines, eating habits, etc. It is also fun to be honest with yourself. When I was writing down that I was starting my day at 10 AM and I saw that I missed 5 hours of potential success and it made me realize that I couldn't use the excuse that there wasn't enough time in a day to be who I wanted to be and at the end of the day we created time, we can change time, we can decide how much of it is in our day. If we wanted to stay awake for 48 hours and then sleep 4 hours you could do that. Now you probably won't be as productive as sleeping when you are tired and getting up when you are full of energy, but you have the control of how you use your time. It will be different for everyone. You may have kids or a job that is an hour drive to get to or it may have weird hours and there will be sacrifices. You may have to get a new job if it's not healthy for you. You know what I mean? If you are using the excuse of time and that you can't make it then you might actually have to tell your boss that this job is to much and you need to dedicate more time for your health so that you have more time with your kids because every day you are closer to being dead. Every day the people that you love are closer to being dead and we have no idea what is after this life. So I hope you make the best choices for your time.

A great application you can download on your smart phone that will help you understand what your body needs on a daily basis is called MyFitnessPal. You can also login through your web browser on your computer. There are many applications to choose from, but this is just one that I have personally used that I have found to help me a lot with the nutrition side of things. In this application you put in your height, age, weight, male or female and then you put in your goal of where you would like to be. Whether you would like to lose 5 pounds or gain 10 pounds and if you would like to lose the weight or gain the weight a pound a week or a half pound, etc. Make the goal realistic and healthy. Take your time losing the weight or gaining it because you can cause a lot of health issues if you do it incorrectly.

It would drive me nuts when I would have clients coming to see me saying they are doing the ketogenic diet and their doctor or dietician gives them this bull shit response of how it is healthy because you starve yourself in a different way where your body won't respond to storing more body fat because you don't eat until 2pm or something insane. You can talk to me about these ridiculous health trends but the bulk of them are not healthy. It is people creating a business model and marketing it to people who don't ask questions. Always ask questions, question everyone, question me, question yourself, question everyone because everyone is doing everything for a reason. I am making this book because I like making money. I also like helping people, but more importantly I am making sure my own personal wellbeing is being taken care of. I like traveling and I found that when I created sources of income that I didn't have to exchange my time for money it freed up my time and I was able to have more success in other areas of my life. I had more time with my friends and family, I was able to travel and I was able to accomplish other things. Just remember to always question people and research my information. No one is one hundred percent correct. It's not on purpose but there are always new studies, new trend, new ideas and I am always striving to better myself and I am constantly trying to give the best information in my books, blogs and videos but no one is going to know everything.

Before you say "Oh well I guess I can't trust anyone, I can't trust Pat…he's a fucking dick. He wrote a book to make money." No, what I am trying to say is learn from people with experience. Learn from people who have what you want, but don't only take their perspective. Be ready to learn from a lot of people, but always check your sources and understand fully of why you are doing what you are doing. Figure out what works for you, start small and be consistent.

If you have a hard time drinking a glass of water then instead of getting an ounce of water per pound of body weight start out by getting a half gallon each day or half your body weight depending on which ever one is an easier goal to obtain. I was reading this blog a few months ago about this lady and how the only thing she changed in her lifestyle was drinking a lot of water throughout the day and she ended up losing 10 lbs. in one month. She didn't exercise and she didn't change anything about her diet besides drinking more water and she was able to see astonishing results.

We tend to forget the basics like drinking lots of water, getting 6 to 8 hours of good sleep, not stressing about stupid shit, staying active and eating fairly well. Fairly well means eating pizza once a week but not being an asshole about it and eating a whole pizza. I am talking about a couple slices. Consistency is the key to success in anything. I will say this often in this book, but it is true. Take a second and think about anything that you are great at. You probably created some sort of consistency that established results and return gave you success. Do you have a college degree? You didn't just get a college degree, you put consistent work in and then you got your degree. Let's say you don't have a college degree, let's say you don't even have a high school diploma, and let's just say you are really good at videos games. You had to consistently turn on your video game system and you had to practice and eventually you became good because you practiced. I didn't say this would be easy, but if you bring consistency to the table then eventually it will be easy. Start by waking up as a winner and doing something good for your body, for your mind and then everything else will fall into place and bring happiness into your life.

When I wake up I like moving around right away. I don't necessarily mean go to the gym, but I do some push-ups or I go for a walk or I bounce on my mini trampoline because it will wake up your body. It will release endorphins, dopamine and other chemicals throughout your body naturally. Instead of paying pharmaceutical drug companies a whole bunch of money to shoot your body up with these chemicals unnaturally and possibly give your body health problems later on down the road.

What you need to do is make sure that you're drinking water immediately when you wake up. Your body is dehydrated. You've been sleeping for 6 to 8 hours hopefully and because of that your body needs liquids. Make this the first priority of your day, along with eating breakfast. Some people will say they don't do breakfast or that they don't eat right when they wake up. I personally think it's important to eat breakfast because that will give you energy for the day and just like the water you haven't had any food for 6 to 8 hours and from the research that I have found is that getting food right when you wake up will kick start your metabolism and get everything going. Think of it as when you start your car in the morning during a cold winter morning and the car is freezing. You have to turn it on and wait a little bit for it to get warm. I believe that is similar to how our bodies work.

Create a system in your life where you're drinking water right when you wake up and immediately before bedtime. Have that morning ritual and nightly routine and in just a matter of weeks that single system change could make a huge difference. It's the little things that we do on a consistent basis that make the big things happen in our life. After, you make sure to start drinking enough water throughout the day then do a self-audit with your life. Be honest with yourself, no one is perfect there is always room for improvement. There are times where I get consistent on drinking coffee with cream and sugar and if I do that long enough then I will eventually pay the price especially if there are artificial sweeteners in my coffee which I would never dare to do. It is all about balance though. Make sure you are happy because stress is a huge factor in weight gain.

When you drink water it helps to hydrate your entire body. You need a lot of water. You should be getting a half an ounce to an ounce of water per pound of body weight. That's how much water (in ounces) that you need to drink each day. If you drink that much your entire body is going to feel better. You're going to feel happier, healthier and you're going to look a lot better as well. That's because your skin cells are some of the last to actually receive hydration. That means you're going to have dry skin as well as dry hair if you're not getting enough water. You also might have more headaches or health problems with less water in your system.

So when you're trying to get your weight under control and you're looking to get more toned you'll be able to do a whole lot just by drinking plenty of water. The more you can drink in a day the better you're going to feel and definitely the healthier you're going to be as well.

Make sure that you drink some water before each of your meals. That will make it so much easier to get your recommended amount of water. For example someone who is 150 pounds needs 75 to 150 ounces of water a day. If you are not at your goal weight you're probably are not getting enough water in your system. If you are getting enough water then that is great news because that means you are one step closer to getting the body you want for yourself. Getting the recommended amount of water for your body weight will also make it easier to eat smaller portions throughout the day and it will be easier to detoxify your body. If you drink more water throughout the day this is also going to reduce how much you eat and how hungry you even feel. And still, cutting a lot of calories out of your daily diet is only one of the many different things that you will be able to achieve when you start adding a lot more water to your diet.

Now that I say that though make sure you are not restricting your calories to low because for most people they aren't eating enough. They may just be drinking 10 beers a night and eating a pint of ice cream before bed and can't comprehend what the fuck happened. If you are eating 3000 calories of vegetables a day instead of 3000 calories of McDonalds you will see completely different results between the two. Don't worry too much about over eating. Just make sure everything is in moderation. If you want pizza, have a slice. Just don't eat the whole pie. If you have a day that you slip up get over it. Don't have a pity party. Just realize what you did and fix it for the future. Eat lots of fruits and vegetables, drink lots of water, get a good source of protein throughout the day so your body can build muscle and minimize your body fat percentage and along with that add healthy fats to your diet so that you protect your heart but also help your physical and emotional health.

A simple morning routine breakfast could include oatmeal and a scoop of protein in your oatmeal. Very simple but this way you're getting a slow digestive carb to have energy right when you wake up and a good source of protein to fuel your muscles and to build your muscle much quicker. If you have a diet that is high in phytic acid just remember brush your teeth and floss like a mad man because oatmeal and cereal can be dangerous and detrimental to your teeth.

Nutrition is the most important aspect, then exercising, then doing the little things and if you're doing all of that then you can add natural supplements to speed up the process. There is no magic pill but if you're doing all the right things than it can definitely help speed up the process of lowering your body fat percentage and building your muscle at a faster rate.

Before you get into supplements though train your brain to believe the basics are supplements. Every time you drink water you are taking Hydroxycut or every time you eat a healthy delicious meal you are doing the Atkins diet. Some scientists did a study on actual diets and it didn't matter what diet the person was doing, but that they were consistent and believed in the diet that gave them the results. Our brains are super powerful. If you can get your mind right and do the small things consistently you will eventually see the results with your body. It's hard to think that you will have to stay accountable with yourself but if you can be consistent, if you can surround yourself with healthy people, get in the same gym as the people you want to look like or play the same sport as them or do some of the same habits as them you will see results.

Before we get into all of that though remember to eat breakfast and to drink water. Another helpful tip can be to take out one negative habit for 14, 21 or 31 days while you add these two positive systems into your life. Just one though, it could be soda, fast food, beer, cream in your coffee. Whatever you may be doing that isn't the healthiest thing for your body. Try taking a break for up to 31 days. Don't try to fix everything though because no one is perfect but if you can eliminate one bad thing and add lots of water, a good simple breakfast and you will be amazed by the results you could possibly get and you will feel really good. You're going to feel better, you're going to look better and if you're working out you will perform better. I guarantee it!

Example of my morning ritual and nightly routine is below.

Morning Ritual

- **Smile…Laugh if you can!**
- **Stretch! (Think of Rinsing a Wet Rag…What comes out? Things that shouldn't be on the rag!)**
- **Meditation/Priming (Give yourself 10 minutes…if you can't have 10 minutes to yourself then you need to fix something.)**
- **Move the body around (Push-ups, Squats, Bounce around on my mini trampoline)**
- **Drink 32 ounces of Water!**
- **Eat Breakfast! (Good source of carbohydrates will give you energy and a good source of protein will help build muscle)**
- **Affirmations (I have these Affirmation cards…You can make your own)**
- **3 Things to be Grateful for (Reduces Stress)**

- **Plan out Your Day! (Without a plan you can't succeed)**
- **Do the most important thing immediately after planning. Do not wait or you will fail.**

Examples of things that I would be accomplishing for the day could be working out, reading 10 pages of a book that will make me smarter and the third could be something to improve a business of mine or it could include be improving a relationship. Remember to strive for balance in your life. I usually stick with 3 things and then when I finish those I will write down whatever else is on my mind and then go do it.

Nightly Routine

- **Make Sure "To Do List" Was Complete! (Helps track Progression)**
- **Pat myself on the Back for what I Completed! (You Have to celebrate your successes…even the small successes)**
- **Be Thankful (Because eventually I will be gone and you will be too!)**
- **Drink 32 ounces of Water! (Got to Stay Hydrated)**
- **If I eat before bed, make it Healthy! (Can't be hungry going to bed just make sure it's healthy)**

Importance of Sleep

Getting plenty of sleep is crucial for your body and mind to recover. The reason is simple. During sleep your body works to repair the muscle that you've worked on through the day. What you may not know is that in order for you to build up more muscle the old muscle has to tear and be rebuilt. Now this is NOT the same as when your doctor says you have a torn muscle. These are very minor tears that are easily repaired overnight by your body. When your doctor tells you that you have a torn muscle (which can happen when you push yourself too hard and too fast) it does not heal that easily and it is a much more serious matter.

During sleep your body creates any of the cells it needs to heal you from the day and your brain is able to rest as well. While the brain is resting it's preparing for the next day. If it doesn't get the rest that it needs in order to prepare, you will wake up groggy, tired and possibly even sick or with a headache the next morning. You definitely don't want any of those things. They're going to result in you being a lot less productive throughout the day and you're definitely going to feel less capable of achieving anything because you won't have enough energy. All of these things are built into your brain while you're sleeping.

Now for an adult the ideal amount of sleep is about 8 hours. Of course, what you really want is for your body to wake up entirely on its own. That means you want to try and wake up without an alarm. This is not always going to be possible. Some people simply don't wake up on their own even when their body has plenty of sleep. If you sleep for 10-12 hours and still wake up groggy that means your body is actually getting too much sleep. The problem is that your body doesn't wake itself up when you're ready to get up and that can result in the same problems that not enough sleep can cause.

Now for most people you're going to need to go to bed earlier in order to make sure you're getting enough sleep. This is because, most adults are not able to sleep in later than they do because of work, family, children, chores or anything else that needs to be done around the house. Figure out a way to get to bed a little earlier and help your body to reenergize itself for the day ahead by getting the right amount of sleep. This is going to help your entire body feel better which makes it easier to lose weight and/or to burn fat.

For me seven hours is usually the magic number. I like to get ready for bed at 9pm and usually fall asleep by 10 PM and by 5 AM my body is ready for the day. It's consistent for the most part excluding vacations and some weekends but that is what works for me. I turn off all electronics except for my alarm clock. I like using an alarm clock though because I've programmed my mind to get excited for it. Most people get a negative reaction from an alarm. What you can do is either A find the time that is best for you to not need an alarm or B during the day when you're wide awake go to your bed, set an alarm for a minute ahead and pretend to go to sleep. When you hear the alarm wake up and get excited. Do this for a few weeks and eventually you can reprogram your brain to be happy when you hear your alarm early in the morning. Eventually you'll feel like a kid and its Christmas morning and you'll run out of bed and kick ass for the day.

Chapter Two

Eliminate Stress

Another huge reason for people not being able to reach their weight goal or reduce their body fat percentage is because their life is a living hell. Stress is the worst thing in the world but there are ways to keep it from controlling your life. I truly believe if you can reduce your stress you will see that your body will be able to get faster results. What I have found that has worked for me to keeping my stress levels at a minimum is that I am very goal oriented. You may say well hey I have goals why am I stressed? Are you accomplishing your goals? Are your goals balanced? Do you have a realistic deadline for yourself to accomplishing your dreams? Are you enjoying process? Or are you rushing success and turning it into failure?

Obviously since you're reading this book you know health and fitness matter to you. This is great news because that means you are ready to make a change in your life! You probably want to lose 10 lbs. or put on some muscle and look like Channing Tatum or you want date someone that looks like Channing Tatum. So since building muscle or burning fat is what is on your mind right now what would you like to see happen with your body? Write it down and be so specific to what you want to accomplish in your life and body.

Then break that down and figure out what you can accomplish today. What do you have control over? Maybe you can run a mile and time it and then the next day you beat that time or you go to the gym and you do a total body workout and you figure out your personal best in the amount of weights or reps you can do and you record it and you keep on gradually getting better. Exercise will definitely help lower stress but don't forget about all the other areas in your life. Make sure you feel balanced with your career or family goals and make progress every day. If you're developing your mind and body each day and you stay in a constant state of gratitude you'll see that your stress will lower over time.

Figure out the things that are stressing you out and make a game plan to get rid of that stress. If you feel tired all the time then give yourself time for sleep. You don't have to exercise every day. You can have days off, but be sure your nutrition is a little better on those days that aren't as active. I have weeks that I work out 5 days a week or 2 days a week or sometimes I even go on vacation. What I do is I limit my stress and if I am anxious about anything then it's usually because I need to do something in my life. I have to make some sort of progress in a certain area. It is usually something I know I am capable of completing in a short amount of time, but whether it is pure laziness or the fear of failure I don't do it. I rarely see those days now because when you start getting a little bit of success you can't stop. It becomes very addicting.

My mind is saying "Hey Pat you said you wanted to do this with your life…Why aren't you doing it?" and then I go and do it and I feel so much better. Don't get stressed out if you're not seeing results fast enough because you probably won't. There is a good chance that this experience is going to be so difficult and you're going to want to quit. When you get those feelings of wanting to quit, think about how you would feel if you succeeded. If everything eventually came together and your conquered your dreams. How would you feel? What would the success be like? Imagine that success that you are about to attract to yourself.

You have a plan. You have that big dream. That ultimate goal in life where you have everything you want and you're not going to quit. You are going to stay in a constant state of gratitude because you're so happy for what you already have and you're so determined to get that dream body and to live the life you've always wanted because you will finally allow yourself to accept the dreams that you constantly think about.

You are not depressed anymore because you're enjoying the process of life. It's okay that you're not at the weight you want to be at or that you're not the strongest person in the room because that would be dumb if life was that easy. What would be the point of life if it was like a video game and you were playing it on easy and you beat it in 5 seconds? You'd be like this bull shit I want my money back. Enjoy the failures, enjoy the success, and get excited for more abundance in your life. It sounds silly but if you can do the little things right and stay happy it will make the process so much easier. You're going to accept this stressful challenge and beat it in the face. It will be so hard, but each day that you make even a little bit of progress you're going to be so excited because you know that you are one day closer to that dream body.

We always want to improve. Make sure each day you're doing that because it's important. Pretend for a moment that your life is a movie and you can do whatever you want. Make this movie the most ultimate movie ever to be made where people are remaking your movie because it was that good. You are winning awards for this movie. You are getting best actor and director because you are the Rocky Balboa of your movie!

Chapter Three

Daily Goals, Systems and Routines

We were just talking about getting enough sleep, drinking water, eating breakfast and lowering stress levels. When you want to succeed at life you need to have rituals or systems built into your world that will make your long term goals come to fruition. Whether it's financial or fitness dreams you need to have a plan and a daily system that will help you succeed.

When I wake up at 5am in the morning I have a big smiling grin on my face and I go into the mirror and I make myself laugh. So that right when I wake up I can be in a constant state of gratitude. After that I chug my 32 ounces of water and eat my breakfast with a couple other things in my morning ritual. Do not stress about having the perfect rituals, just understand there has to be some consistency in your day to day habits. I also like to include different little health trends like a shot of Wheat Grass or Apple Cider Vinegar. At one point I was eating an egg shell a day to whiten my teeth and to get a load of calcium and minerals so that they could be naturally stronger.

Do your research. Figure out what is going to work for you. I am always looking to improve myself. Do the little things right, like eating the right foods, not getting down on yourself when you mess up, but understanding and growing from that experience. Drinking lots of water, getting a good amount of sleep, saying thank you to people every chance you get, listening to people, consistently being active. When you wake up you should be excited. Pretend it is Christmas morning when you were a kid and if Christmas was never an exciting holiday for you then think of a day or a time that it was just perfect.

Everything was right and if you can visualize that excitement for every day that you get to have for the rest of your life because eventually you are going to die. You will die, I will die, your parents will die, your friends will die, your brothers and sisters will die, everyone is going to die and we don't really know what happens when we "die" so we might as well make this life our heaven. I don't mean to stress you out, but you need to wake up. If there are things in your life that make you sad or depressed or angry or upset then you need to wake your ass up because no matter how hard it is you still have it better then someone else. It is okay to have a pity party every now and then, but don't be known for it. Don't let too many people know that you get down because then they will look down on you and no one wants that. You don't want people to feel sorry for you. If you have people feeling sorry for you then chances are you don't have a significant other, people might think you're crazy or emotionally unstable and it's not fair for them to judge you like that, but you cannot blame them for wanting too! I bet you can think of a multiple occasions where you just judged the shit out of someone because they were either annoying, or their ideas sucked, or they just sucked to be around, they were just so freaking emotional and draining where all you wanted to do was get the fuck out.

Think of one person in your life who is just so amazing to be around. They are funny, smiling, uplifting, always encouraging, always learning, always bettering themselves and if you honestly don't have anyone like that in your life then look to people on the internet or in books like Robin Sharma, Tony Robbins, Jim Rohn, Will Smith, Ray Lewis or invest in a coach or a personal trainer. Invest your money in yourself. Especially if you are finding that every day you are spending $3.33 on your mocha frappe that is loaded with sugar and calories when at the end of the month that is $99.90 that could easily pay for a single session with someone who has what you want. People are so afraid to invest in themselves. I've spent thousands and thousands of dollars on coaches and trainers and people that I wanted to surround myself with because I knew if I did then I would be able to eventually have what they had.

Find the things that work for you and excite your morning. If you're not waking up like a power house everyday then you're doing something wrong. Your mind has to be in the right place to deserve what you want outwardly. After I wake up, hydrate myself, give myself the nutrition my body needs and do some of the health trends I'm interested in. I create a game plan of three things I want to accomplish for the day.

The reason I stick with three daily goals is because it's easy to accomplish and it doesn't overwhelm me where I'm able to accomplish all three and then if I have more time in the day then I can go back to the drawing boards and figure out what else needs to be accomplished or if I'm satisfied then it gives me the opportunity to relax or to reward myself in some other way.

You might be asking yourself how is this going to give me that flat stomach or those chiseled abs. Well if none of your goals for the day are geared towards fitness then this won't, but if you create a morning ritual where when you wake up you tell yourself or you write down in your journal that you're going to hit the gym for 45 minutes and do 30 minutes of high tempo exercise with your gym buddy or your personal trainer and fifteen minutes of intense cardio and it's your goal to decrease the time of your mile by 15 seconds then yes this morning ritual will definitely help you succeed and get you that sexy body you've always been looking for.

You can't stop at just writing it down. You have to commit yourself to accomplishing your fitness goals. What I personally like to do is every now and then I write down my six month and yearly goals for everything from my fitness and health to my financial and travel goals. Then I figure out what is realistic for me to accomplish for these dreams in the short amount of time like within this month, the next two weeks and today. I try to keep it balance. If you're only focused on your health chances are your relationships aren't the greatest because you're just posting gym selfies on the internet and not listening to the person that is hoping for your relationship. Think of a couple long term fitness goals you would like to achieve like train for a marathon and complete it or compete in a local cross fit competition and place in the top 3. Maybe it's realistic for you to win a body building competition or to walk on to a college football team, but find the things that are realistic to accomplish in a year from now and have some short term goals that relate to it that you can accomplish within the next 90 days.

You can do this with all types of goals just make sure they're realistic to how your life is now. You may be 300 pounds right now and you can't even walk a mile without your joints hurting. So your year goal might be to lose 30 pounds, to improve your flexibility and range of motion and be able to run a mile in under 18 minutes.

Once you have your goals set in place make a daily system that you can implement into your life that will actually help you succeed with your goals. Take a moment and think about something that you're talented at or your pretty good at. How much work or time had to be invested to reach that greatness or to complete that task or to get that degree? You will have to implement things in your life that need to be repeated.

You're not going to get shredded abs if you eat a bowl of ice cream every night before bed and drink sugary drinks and please do not drink diet soda or anything that says sugar free or fat free. Chances are it's loaded with artificial sweeteners that expand into your body and create more room for fat to be loaded into your system. As well as countless studies that say these fake ingredients are the root cause for all these deadly diseases like diabetes, heart disease, cholesterol issues and the list goes on. It hurts my heart when I see people coming in for a consultation and their bodies are so out of whack and it's from their own consistent doing. Things that they did consistently to the point where they are almost dead and I don't blame them because sometimes we are not educated on everything that we need to be educated on, but it is scary. You wonder what they are dealing with emotionally and physically. Life is hard. I understand that and I can sympathize with you if you don't have the body you want. I've been there when I was in high school and was the little guy and when I lost 40 lbs. in twenty days when I was in the hospital for my Crohns diagnosis. It can break you down and there will be times when you feel like you got nothing left in you, but I'm telling you if you are still breathing and you have even the slightest hope for a better future, you can make it happen.

Look at yourself in the mirror and ask yourself honestly are you doing everything perfectly with your nutrition? How about your activity level? Are you running a mile a day or doing a strength training program or even playing with your kids for 60 minutes a day? What are your current daily systems in your life? Your friend Jenny might have the "perfect body" but doesn't do anything. Don't worry about what she's doing. If you put the work in then you will see the results. Start small get a gym membership, walk a mile. Then the next day go in and make that mile a little bit faster. Do it again and again until your body can't get faster. Pick up a weight and lift it. Then lift a little bit heavier of a weight and keep on adding weight until you can't add any more weight, do more reps, less rest, make the tempo more difficult. Whatever you have to do to get what you want, then you must do it because you only have one life. If everyone thought of their body as they do with money, the world would be a much healthier place.

Set small attainable goals for the beginning, but have that vision in your mind with that perfect body that you picture and wish for every day. You can do this, but if you don't have that perfect vision of your life and you can't believe it can happen then it will never come true. Quit letting your excuses control your life. God put you in this world for a reason and he gave you these dreams and aspirations for a purpose. He's making it hard because you will appreciate it when you succeed. He's putting you through these trials and tribulations to make you better. No one wants to play a video game on "Easy" because it takes the fun out of it and you can't really be proud of beating something that is letting you win. You have to take it! You have to make what you want to come true.

Right now you deserve exactly what you have. Change your perspective; create healthy habits and systems in your life! You can make anything happen but your mind is a battleground and you have to make war with it to accomplish your dreams.

Chapter Four

Surround Yourself with the Greats

If you are really serious about getting healthy your best option is to surround yourself with experts. When I was 15 and 90 pounds I surrounded myself with friends that were strong and had the body that I wanted. It was hard at first. I don't think I really saw much in the first year because I would get discouraged and I would cry and moan to my parents that they made me this way, but they didn't. I decided to do that with my actions and continuous habits. I was the one who picked the video games or the television over a consistent workout regimen because I was scared. I was scared to work, I already had to get good grades, I was already playing sports and I thought I was already doing enough, but sometimes you have to look past your own understandings and seek smarter people.

Luckily something came within me and I decided to make a change. I decided that enough was enough. I made my goal so specific and I trained with my strong friends and before bed I would do push-ups and sit-ups until I couldn't do anymore because I was determined to make a change. I trained so hard and every 30 days I would post a new picture up on Myspace and I told myself every day I'm almost there. I had the attitude I needed to have success. I would have never gotten results if I didn't surround myself with people that believed in me or were at least willing to help me and give me advice on what I needed to do. The reason I made that reference to Myspace is because this journey started a long time ago and hopefully for the rest of my life it will be a lifestyle of mine. This can't be temporary and it doesn't have to be a gym facility you can create this lifestyle with so many different avenues. Find the things that you enjoy but also don't be scared to try new things. We're creatures of habit and we gravitate to what we're comfortable with.

If you want to succeed find someone that has what you want and talk to them, ask them questions and figure out what you have to do. I do this with every area of my life. When I wasn't financially free I went to business owners and people that were living millionaire lifestyles and I asked them questions and did what they said. I bought coaching for my businesses. When I was in high school I went to the football players and aspiring body builders. I went to the people who knew what they were doing and repeated their actions that I found useful.

Be honest (at least in your own mind), how many times have you decided that you were going to start exercising, get in shape and lose weight and then stopped? How many times did you start out strong and then end up falling right back into your old ways? If you're like the rest of us (myself included) more times than you can count.

The problem is that you didn't have anyone counting on you in those instances. No one was waiting for you to show up at the gym or to present your food log. You had no one but yourself to be accountable to and you ended up giving yourself a pass. You let yourself just slide and decided that the lifestyle wasn't worth it. Maybe you figured it was too difficult or maybe you only meant to have one day be a skip day and ended up falling off the wagon entirely. It happens to the best of us.

What you need is a mentor or a trainer because they will keep you accountable. If you have a partner that expects you to show up at a specific time to work out or to go to a class that you're expected to attend you feel obligated to go even if you don't want to. You feel like someone is depending on you and that makes you more inclined to do it. Maybe you even convince yourself that you're doing it for other people. Whatever works for you!

You want to choose someone that's really going to motivate you as well. If you pick a friend that you can easily call up and say 'I'm just not feeling it today' and they'll say 'okay, maybe tomorrow' you're not helping each other. This type of conversation and fitness relationship is not going to motivate you. What you need is a partner that is going to help you become an unstoppable force. Find someone or talk to a person today that is educated in health and fitness, but who is not only educated but also lives a lifestyle that you can see on their body. Don't call your friend Frank who drinks 18 beers a night and has this cool kick ball underneath his shirt.

Go to your gym and see who is a personal trainer there. Find the one that you think you would match up well with. I bet if you go into your gym there will probably be bios on all the trainers at your gym. If there is not then they are losing out on a lot of potential clients, but more than likely they do. Read them and see whose expertise seems right for you. Look at the trainers who have a lot of clients, look at their clients, are they progressing.

I may be biased, but I would look for a trainer who has a lot of personality, someone who likes to listen and actually understand you. I think I was more of a therapist when I was a full time trainer, but I loved it and I was very good at coaching. I was able to get anybody results because I understood how to relate to people. Do not go for the trainer who is book smart, who knows the most terminology, find the trainers who are dedicated to you and making sure you get the results you want because at the end of the day the trainer is suppose be there for you. If they are on their iPad to look more professional and trying to scheme you run. Find a trainer who doesn't have technology on them, find a trainer who uses a pen and paper. Don't expect them to do everything though. If you would like to impress your coach come there ready with your own pen and journal and ready to go. Write down everything because eventually you'll be the teacher. You don't want to be the student forever. Hopefully you can gain a lot of knowledge and then pass that on to someone you care about. Maybe you eventually start seeing results and your husband wants to get in the gym as well. You guys could either do partner training or if you have built up enough knowledge and confidence you two could work together, but make sure you are ready.

I still at times get coaches for my own training. I am physically fit, but I love learning and knowing more than everyone else. It's in my fucking gene pool to be a genius.

In the meantime I created a Facebook group for people to join where we can keep each other accountable on our health and fitness goals called *Make Life Your Body*. In this group we give each other advice, positive encouragement towards each other's dreams and goals for our health and fitness. If you have friends and family that are struggling, anyone can join. I personally try and reach out to everyone that is in the group and see if there is any way that I can personally help.

We are steadily growing and we have a lot of very experienced athletes, coaches and people that have incredible fitness journeys and if we have people who are just starting out or getting back into. We are all helping each other become better. It's free to join so you might as well come aboard and learn or teach if you have experience in the health and fitness industry.

Chapter Five

Challenge Yourself

I love to dare myself or to challenge my body and mind. Whether it's a body cleanse or I give up something that I may be focusing on that probably isn't the healthiest thing in my life. I'm a normal human being. I like to have fun, I make mistakes, I live and I learn.

One of my favorite things to give up is alcohol. I'm going to be honest, beer tastes very good, hanging out with friends is fun and cracking a cold one is always a good time, but you know what else is cool? Changing something drastic in your life and seeing what happens. You learn a lot about yourself. You may already be alcohol free or under the age to drink, but maybe you love fast food and you can't get enough of it. Try giving it up for 31 days or even 14 days or 21 days and see how your body feels.

We're creatures of habit. It usually takes about 21-66 days to break a habit so you might even find that whatever you were doing with your life before you might not even feel like going back to it. You might build up this phenomenal taste for a clean and healthy lifestyle. You might dare yourself first to give up alcohol and then you go to doing a paleo lifestyle or a vegan lifestyle. It might be as simple as not going out to eat and saving money and cooking your own food.

Dare yourself and give yourself a deadline to when you can finish the dare. Do something that your body would be so confused, but at the same time thanking you for taking care of it. There are so many things that we abuse on a consistent basis and they're the biggest red flags to why our health isn't where it needs to be. So dare yourself and be a freaking bad ass!

You'll find that if you do these challenges your health will sky rocket, but not only will your body transform into the figure you desire, but your wealth will start to build, your mind will start to grow, you'll start finding more balance in your life and because of that you'll start to have more confidence. If you are having trouble thinking of something to give up I will list some of my favorites.

Challenge List (Give up)
- Alcohol
- Tobacco
- Television
- Fast food
- Energy drinks
- Sweet tea
- Diet soda
- Video games
- Bread
- Cream and sugar in your coffee

Challenge List (Create Habit)
- Drink half ounce to an ounce of water per pound of body weight a day
- Walk or run every day
- Eat breakfast within 30 minutes of waking up
- Drink black coffee or bullet proof coffee
- Go to the gym 3 days a week
- Shot of wheat grass every morning
- Get 6 to 8 hours of sleep a night
- Journal your workouts
- Use MyFitnessPal application to track what you're eating
- Squat Challenge. Squat every day and do at least one more rep than the day before.

Chapter Six

Have a Vision, Collect Data and Progress

Food Journal!

If you want to understand why you are or aren't losing weight you need to start a food journal. This is a place to write down absolutely everything that you eat at any period during the day. You want to keep it with you at all times so that means you want something small that's going to be easy to carry either in your purse/bag or your back pocket. This journal should go with you everywhere and it should come out after everything that you eat. That's the only way you can make sure you're tracking everything. If you don't want to have a note pad with you try downloading an application on your phone that will track your food.

You may be thinking, I could just write everything down when I get home. You could if you had an eidetic memory (that means you remember absolutely everything that happens to you ever). Unfortunately, an extremely small percentage of the world has an eidetic memory. That means you will find yourself forgetting that one soda from the break room or the few crackers you picked up on your way to work. Every little thing needs to be written down because otherwise you could find yourself struggling to lose weight and not knowing why it's happening or what you need to do in order to stop it.

The first thing to do is work on your food journal before you even start to a new lifestyle. Write everything you eat or drink from the moment you get up until the moment you go to bed. Try to get a good estimate on the size of the item as well. So a 12 oz. Coke instead of 'soda.' Or 5 cheese crackers instead of just 'crackers.' You want to be as specific as possible so that later you can go through and figure out the total number of calories, carbs, fats and proteins you're actually eating in a normal day. You'll be able to see how much you really need to cut out and/or add to your meals.

Most people think they need to cut out calories but for most you're not eating enough throughout the day so your body stores more fat. The reason it stores more fat is because it's confused that it's not getting the proper nutrition. In some cases you may be over eating. It may be calories but usually it's a macro like Carbohydrates or you're getting all your carbs from pastas and breads and not fruits and vegetables. I'm not saying you can't eat pizza ever again but make everything in moderation. If you're working out and you pushed yourself to the limits and burned 1000 calories then have a piece of cake, but remember to add some good stuff in your day.

I personally like the 80/20 rule because stress is probably the biggest factor to people gaining weight and not being able to achieve the body they want. I focus on all the good things I'm doing for my body. If I'm getting my shot of wheat grass, drinking tons of water, exercising on a daily basis, eating lots of vegetables, fruits and lean meats then I don't feel bad when I have a piece of cake at my niece's birthday party or if I want to have a pizza party I'll smash a couple slices. Everything in moderation and reward yourself when your crushing life and never consider it a "diet" this is your lifestyle

Exercise Journal

The next thing you want to do is start an exercise journal. This is where you're going to write down every time that you exercise each day. Now you don't want to include 'walking to the break room' or 'walked to the car.' These are not really going to burn a lot of calories (unless you walked to the break room down the street or you parked your car a mile from work). They are also not really going to be considered 'exercise' in this sense (again unless the mentioned circumstances apply). You want to count times when you actively decided you were going to exercise.

So if you went to the gym for twenty minutes on the treadmill write it down. Write down that you walked around your block for ten minutes or jogged in place for 15 minutes and between every 20 seconds you did 5 body squats. Those things are exercise and they are helping you to burn some calories as well. When you make yourself more accountable for your exercise it works in two different ways. The first is that you see how much you are exercising already and you feel proud of yourself for the accomplishments you've made. The other is you realize you're not exercising enough and decide to work a little harder.

Also, when you can look at the amount of exercise that you're actually getting you're going to feel better about yourself as well because you can see the amount of work that you're producing. This is going to improve your opinion of yourself and improve your opinion about the exercise program you're working on. By recording everything you do, you make it easier to keep track of how close you are to the goals that you've set for yourself and to achieving everything you really want from your weight loss and body transformation journey.

Change it up. Don't make yourself feel that you have to be at a gym facility every week. Maybe you go on a summer beach vacation. You can run a mile on the beach and do some sunrise yoga a couple days during your vacation. Maybe you and the family go on an outside family adventure to a park and throw a Frisbee around or play a game of kickball. In my opinion I believe we should just be as active as possible and adventuring in this world. I don't believe anyone should be stuck in 9 to 5 jobs sitting the whole day, finding out they have hip pain and then coming home and being too tired to do anything.

Enjoy your one life that you get because as far as we know this is the only one we get so make the best out of it. Be creative, be happy, enjoy life and exercise your mind and body! When you start this adventure just remember to record everything to keep yourself accountable and to look back on it. It will seem hard at first, but after a year it will be all worth it if you stayed consistent in your new healthy habits. Embrace the pain, the struggles, the stress, the hard work and be happy that you are now a bad ass at life.

Set Goals and Deadlines

I mentioned this a little bit earlier but I want to go more in depth. I find it very important to create performance goals to succeed in life. If you want your body to be ready for the beach then what goals do you have for yourself?

I always have goals and a timetable for when I want to accomplish my dreams or when I believe it's realistic for me to complete the aspirations I have for myself. Start with the unrealistic things first. The things that would take a few years, then from there what do you think you could complete in 12 months? From those things you listed that you want to complete in the next year what would need to be completed in 6 months for these goals to maintain their realistic ability to be accomplished. Then from there think of the daily habits and the goals that you have for yourself that need to be completed within the next 90 days and then write them down.

Say you are 250 pounds and in two to three years you would like to be at 18% body fat. You would also like to complete a marathon, a triathlon, compete in a fitness competition and get back into playing soccer on a regular basis. A year from now maybe you make it your goal to get under 200 pounds, you complete a half marathon, you start riding a bike at the gym or outside on a weekly basis and you start swimming on a regular basis at your gym facility or outside if it's warm and to eventually be ready for a fitness competition you get on a strength building program for your body.

Then six months from now you're hoping that based off of your hard work and dedication to these goals you hope that you can be down 25 pounds. You ran your first 5k and you're getting ready for your first 10k. You're riding 10-30 miles a week on your bike and swimming 70 laps a week in your pool.

Then from there you know that today you need to get that gym membership at the facility with the indoor pool because it's getting cold out. You decide to take advantage of a personal trainer because you're ready to invest in your health instead of taking the chance and investing with pharmaceutical drugs because you don't feel like getting diabetes and you don't want high blood pressure!

You are smart! You know that if you have a trainer pushing you and motivating you and getting you on the correct strength program based off your longer term goals it's going to be more realistic to obtain the goals you want to accomplish for your life. You start writing in your journal with all the phenomenal exercises and activities you're doing and you're tracking your nutrition. You find that you're getting a little bit more carbohydrates than you really need so you quickly change a couple daily habits and you're now on track with your meals. Every now and then though you find that your crushing it in the gym and you could have a few hundred more calories for the night so you rent a Redbox with your loved one and have a glass of wine because you know it's time to reward yourself.

Figure out the game plan and the step by steps on accomplishing these goals. Make it realistic, but not too easy. If you want a sexy stomach and smooth legs with no spider webs or cottage cheese figure out some fun goals that you would like to accomplish.

My one friend who had never been to a gym until a year and half ago went from 180 lbs. to 135 lbs. and her body fat went from 41 percent to I believe is now 20% and her journey has just started. She didn't start taking it serious until 7 months ago when she started implementing these systems into her life. She went from being too scared to be at the gym by herself, to training with me one time a week, going to cross fit sessions 2-3 days a week (on her own) and even introducing yoga and other group classes. Now she is more confident than ever. She has signed up for her first cross fit competition in a few months, she's done 5k's and she is constantly branching out and trying new things. She even started taking dance classes and joined a volley ball league.

When I met her and took her to the gym for the first time her attitude was "This is dumb. I don't want to be here." To calling me up and asking me if I want to go on a hike or go trapeze, which I still need to take her up on the trapeze adventure, but I'm deathly scared of heights.

Create a Vision Board

A vision board is something that works for absolutely any goals you have for yourself. Whether you want to run a 5k or you want to travel to France you can use a vision board to help you turn your dreams and goals into something completely real. That's because these boards are intended to help you really see and experience your goal before you ever even get there. After all, you have reason for wanting to run a 5k or travel to France. So use those things to motivate yourself.

Take a magazine and start cutting out pictures of your goals and dreams. Do you see the house that you've always wanted to live in? Cut it out and put it on the board. See the locations you've always wanted to visit? Cut them out and put them on the board. Everything you put on your board should mean something to you. It should either be a dream, a goal or a motivator (or a combination of the three). This board should then go somewhere that you're going to see it every day even without having to go out of your way.

The vision board shows you why you're working so hard. It shows you why you're doing everything that you're doing whether it's working out, saving freedom units aka "money" or just going after career goals. It's your motivation to start working harder at the things you do so that you can make sure you achieve whatever you've set your mind to. You want to just make sure that it's the perfect board for you. Don't let anyone else put things on your board because then it's not going to motive you personally and that's the entire reason that you have it after all.

If you have your vision board, your journal and your mind in the right state it will really help you succeed at a much faster rate. If you have a picture that you can visualize of all the successes in your life it makes it so much easier. Find pictures of that dream body you want or that dream relationship and vacation. Make multiple boards, have multiple journals, get organized and set up these systems in your life.

The reason I'm telling you all these things is because they actually work. I've used these systems from a young age and I have tested it with family and friends and it makes everything achievable. From your fitness level, to your relationships all the way to your business ideas and road to financial freedom, these strategies really work!

White Board

A good thing to set up right next to your vision board is a white dry erase board. I find them very useful with managing your time and completing tasks along with saving paper. I mainly use my white board to schedule my day from 5 AM to 10 PM. If I have appointments or obligations for the day I will write them into their corresponding time frames. This helps me stay organized, reduces stress, gives me a plan of action and allows me to prioritize my personal goals accordingly to what my life has planned for the day.

Set up a white board for however you choose. Sometimes I have it to just write daily a couple daily goals, or quotes or affirmations so that I remind myself of the live that I want for my future.

It may seem like a lot of systems that need to be put in place, but I feel that once I started doing this I was more successful, I was happier, I felt like I had more control and my life has been a huge blessing ever since I got very organized.

Use Technology and Apps!

There are a lot of different apps that are available to those who are trying to reach fitness goals. Some are available on each of the mobile platforms so whether you have a Microsoft Phone, an Android or an Apple or anything in between you'll be able to get some apps that are going to help you be more productive and also help you keep track of what you're eating and what type of exercise you're doing at all times. This is going to make it even easier to reach the goals you've set because you'll have a way of keeping track.

Now some apps are going to help you keep track of exercise simply by acting as a pedometer or a heart rate monitor even. Some are just going to allow you to put information into them and they'll create a chart of the amount of calories you burned and the amount you've taken in. These can tell you how well you're doing as far as sticking to your lifestyle because they'll let you know how much more or less you need to do or eat in order to make sure that you're actually losing body fat and/or gaining muscle instead of staying the same or going in the wrong direction.

Another method you can use is a standard pedometer or heart rate monitor. It will help you understand how many steps you take each day or what your heart rate is at any time. A heart rate monitor is going to tell you when you're exercising strenuously and when you're just sort of pushing yourself. You need to understand your heart rate and how it works best in order to use this method as a way of creating your ideal exercise plan and creating an ideal heart rate to work towards.

The basis you want to use is 220. Take 220 and subtract your current age (such as 30 years old). You'll come to a total of 190 which is then your maximum heart rate. Your desired heart rate for exercise should be between 50 and 85% of that maximum heart rate. Make sure that you don't start out at the top end of this because you're going to push yourself too hard and too fast and you could end up hurt. You want to work your way up to a higher heart rate because that means you're working a lot more and you're burning a lot more calories.

If you're looking for even more ways that you can start burning some calories you should look into a type of fitness band. There are a variety of these and they can keep track of all different things from your calorie intake and output to your heart rate, your exercise and even more. By doing this you'll be able to improve yourself and you'll start losing weight a lot faster because you'll be able to see the great things that you're already doing and the things that you need to do in order to keep losing even more.

Chapter Seven

Importance of Exercise

Possibly one of the most important things you need to do in order to lose body fat is to exercise. Make sure that you're working out all parts of your body and that you're alternating on different parts of your body each day. Spend one day working on your arms or upper body and then spend the next day working on your lower body. By alternating you give the different parts of your body enough time to rest and relax. That means you don't have to worry as much about hurting yourself. That means you give your body time to recover to actually have the opportunity to see results.

You don't have to be in the gym for 3 hours working out like a body builder. There are days where I am just doing a quick 15 minute workout. What you do have to do is be consistent. Don't pick up the habit of exercise for a month or two. Make exercise and healthy habits just a part of your lifestyle. It is what you do. You just can't get enough of it because you love spending time dancing, or going to the gym, or running outside because you love vitamin D. There are so many ways to be physically active.

There is no reason to say you can't do it or that you don't have time. All that you do have is time. If your job says you can't work out then leave! That right there means they don't give a shit about you. Change your perspective in life. Don't allow yourself to be weak. It's okay to be overweight, it's okay to be weak physically, and it's okay to not be good at something.

What is not okay is that you don't do anything about it. Do not let yourself be that person, because you are great and you know you have potential. You know how bad ass you are. It's your time. It's your time to succeed; it's your time to be the person you deserve to be because it's your dream. It is your desire. It is your aspiration. Make it happen!

Surround yourself with the people that see your potential to be great and to achieve what you truly desire for your life. If you feel like the people that you are around bring you down. Guess whose fault that is? Just take a little guess! That's right it's your fault, no one else's! If you have to be by yourself, if you have to shut yourself away from people, if you have to cut people off or cut off certain habits, then do it. Make the fucking change! Make the decision! You already know what you have to do. You already know deep down in the center of your soul what you have to do to be great; to be who God or the Universe needs you to be!

Change your perspective. Fake it until you make it. Do you really think Muhammad Ali was the greatest? He did, He thought he was, I'm sure he had a lot of self-doubt when he was alone at night. I am sure he was running all the ideas of failure in his methodical brain of why he wasn't actually the greatest, but he had to fake it and when he faked it, everyone believed him. Everyone hopped on his wagon, everyone wanted what he had, but guess what he had to fake the idea of being the greatest. He persuaded all of us that he was the greatest boxer of all time.

Now what if you started doing that? Let me tell you a quick story of how believing what you say to yourself can actually give you what you truly want or what you truly don't want. I was working for this company as a personal trainer and I was let go from that company. One of the things management told me was "Patrick you are replaceable." When he said that I agreed and a couple minutes later he let me go. That was the last time I allowed anyone to speak on my behalf and that was the last time I put myself in a situation where I was replaceable. From that day on I put myself first. I told myself I am the greatest. I am talented, unstoppable, one of a kind, intelligent, good looking, hardworking and a good person. I now own multiple online businesses; I travel all over the world, I have spoken in front of thousands of people, I have been able to change a lot of people's lives. I now have so much free time where I am able to do things I am passionate about like acting, stand-up comedy, vacation with my family and friends and the list goes on and on.

What is going to be your story? In life we will either make decisions based off of inspiration or desperation. I have made a lot of decisions using both pathways and neither is wrong, but if you have an ultimate dream that you desire for yourself. If you want to be super strong and defined, you want to travel the world; you want a sexy relationship, you want to be happy and achieve your dreams then believe in yourself! Believe you have it already. When I started doing that my life made a complete 180 for the best. I started getting everything that I wanted out of life. I use to allow my story to be depression, sadness, weak, but now I am great, unstoppable, and hardworking and I continue to dream new dreams and I accomplish them. I set a date, I create plan and then I act on it.

OVERHEAD SQUAT ASSESSMENT

If you are not sure how to set up a workout program and you don't have a personal trainer or coach just yet, you can do a test called an overhead squat assessment. This assessment will let you know what you need to strengthen and stretch based off of what muscles are overactive or underactive. You will need a friend to take a picture of your squat and you want to repeat the squat for about 10 repetitions. What you will need to do is have your feet shoulder width apart, your arms straight up in the air. Your feet will be pointed straight and you will squat down to whatever level you feel comfortable going. You will want your friend to take pictures from the front, side and back. What you will be looking for is compensations within your body. Say your feet turn out or your knees cave in. That is not good and means that you will need to strengthen and stretch certain areas of your body. I would invest in a foam roller and start learning a wide variety of stretches for before and after your workouts so that your body can properly be stretched and strengthen. Remember not to stretch cold muscles, before you stretch make sure you get your body moving either on a bike or treadmill for 5 minutes, you could also do a dynamic workout which includes some stretching, but you are moving at the same time and getting your muscles warmed up.

One on One Coaching

If you are unsure of where to start and would like to receive coaching from myself you can email me at *pwithrow05@gmail.com*. I only coach and train a handful of people because I want to make sure that I am getting my clients great results. Shoot me an email and we can set up an interview time through Skype. If you are someone who quits very easily I will unfortunately not be able to work with you. My time is precious and I only work with people who have a huge desire to succeed. If this is you please email me and we can get started after we have a consultation through Skype.

Chapter Eight

Natural Supplements

You really need to make sure you're getting all the vitamins and minerals that your body needs on a day to day basis. In order to do that you may need to take some supplements for the recommended daily amounts. Keep in mind that the best thing you can do is get all of those vitamins and minerals the natural way. That means through eating fruits, vegetables, fish, nuts, lean mean and other healthy sources of food. This is the way that your body is going to absorb the most nutrients.

It may mean spending a little bit more money on healthier, more nutritious, properly raised meats and natural grown food sources, but then you will end up saving money by not needing to buy prescription drugs that will fuck your life over. Understand that a doctor does not necessarily have more education in your body. He or she is probably very smart, but you should always question what a person's intentions are. My intentions for this book is to help you, but to also make a lot of money through the internet so that I have more time with family and friends and when I train my clients I am doing it because I want to be there not because I need more money. Understand why a doctor may say you need a certain surgery or this prescription. Is he getting a kick back if you use this brand? Just like someone who is an affiliate marketer. He or she is offering you a product because they know if you buy it or buy something because of them they get money.

Always ask questions, our society does not do it enough and we walk blindly in this world too often, but before we get off topic let's keep back to natural supplements!

Some vitamins and minerals are only available to your body through the food you eat and the things you drink. Others you may be able to get reasonably well through a pill supplement. So start by eating a lot of fruits and vegetables. If you still seem to be short on some certain vitamins or minerals go ahead and take a supplement to help you get the right values. There is a very important reason that you get those certain amounts of each vitamin and mineral after all.

Do your research, compare different brands and understand what you're putting in your body and why you are doing it. If you are a female and you notice that your vitamin D and Calcium is low, especially for older women you are more than likely to be deficient in it. Maybe you take your calcium supplement at night because you know it easier to absorb before bed time and because you know it is harder to absorb other vitamins when you take a calcium supplement. There are so many books, so many theories and ideas for anything and everything about life. If you want to be experts on anything read at least 10 books or get 10 different perspectives from people you trust on that one idea and then make up your mind and figure out what you believe. Always question people, where did they get their knowledge. I got my knowledge from tons of trainers, supplement books, coaching books, classes, seminars, internships and much, much, more. You still want to question me though because my answers could be flawed. Everything is flawed, but hopefully you knowing that I know that I am not perfect I am hopefully making you better and ready to crush your goals.

The recommended amounts for each of those vitamins and minerals are important because it allows your body to continue functioning the way that it needs to. For example, some vitamins are required to keep your body producing skin cells in a healthy way. Some produce immunities, some help to send messages through your veins. All of these things are extremely important to the overall function of your body. If you aren't careful and don't get enough of those vitamins or minerals you'll find yourself suffering. Your health will start to decrease and you'll notice that you just don't feel as good as you used to.

Your doctor will be able to tell you if you have any specific vitamin deficiencies. It's important to talk with your doctor before you start taking your own supplements because there are some vitamins that are actually harmful if you take them in too high of quantities based off of some studies. So if you're getting them in your diet and you take a supplement it can actually be a problem for your body. Also, some supplements may interact negatively with medications that you're taking or conditions you may have. Your doctor will be able to help you navigate all these potential problems. I would also recommend seeing multiple doctors for their advice. Their job is just as much as a sales job as it is to look out for your benefit. Always ask questions, watch documentaries on Netflix like Fat, Sick and Nearly Dead and Food Inc. Surround yourself with people who are experienced in nutrition, who are dietitians, personal trainers, people that are passionate about their health and fitness. If your doctor is severely overweight or looks unhealthy then run away find the people who actually live the life they preach to you. Not all medications are bad, but now a day instead of fixing the problem with intelligence we have pharmaceutical drug companies making a killing off of our uneducated individuals in this world. It bullshit, but I guess that's where we got the idea of survival of the fittest.

I was uneducated at one point in my life. I was diagnosed with Crohn's disease and I took doctor's advice to heart. I was told I needed to be medicated to live a healthy life. I didn't ask questions but what happened was I started taking these medications and my health was getting worse. I was getting sick all the time, my body felt weak and it was because I didn't ask questions. I didn't read the bottle that my immune system would be worse if I took this medication. When I finally educated myself, I didn't have Crohn's! I ate hot pockets, drank energy drinks with artificial sweeteners, I drank beer with GMO's, and made poor choices towards my health. What did I think was going to happen? Some of us literally take our day to find the problems instead of just being successful, instead of just progressing, instead of enjoying the process of life. If your one of those people who try to find the problems, who try to find failure then stop reading this book and keep on getting bad results because that is what you want and if that is not what you want then quit the bull shit and be who you need to be!

What you have to understand is a doctor is a person, a person just like you and me. Ultimately you have to ask yourself if what you are doing on a day to day basis is it benefiting you? It's okay not to be perfect, one single decision is not going to determine your life, but a whole bunch of habits that are consistently being done will determine where your life goes. If you make it a priority to get to that drive thru as fast as you can so that you can get that delicious egg sandwich every day and every month and every year you better fucking believe it's going to come after you one day. You are what you eat. You truly know what you are doing is either good or bad for yourself. What is it going to be? How are you going to treat your body today? What questions are you asking? How are you being better each day? Make action today, create healthy habits and after doing the little things right and you feel like you are still having short comings, then yes please take a multivitamin. If you want a fat burner just drink black coffee that will give you the caffeine you need to raise your heart rate which will make you sweat much quicker in the gym. If you want to kill stomach toxins then drink green tea…but just green tea. Do not sweeten that shit. I swear if you tell me you are being healthy and you are drinking diet soda, eating sugar free cookies, and fat free crackers you have another thing coming. You need to educate yourself. I'm not trying to be harsh. You can look up any diet fad or 10 day program to lose 10 pounds but guess what? Life does not work like that. You need to create action and make it a life style. If you are reading this book, then you are capable, you are an adult, you know deep down what you need to change. If it's an addiction to watching hours and hours of television, or scrolling through your Facebook news feed until your fingers bleed then I would start there. That is where I would change something. It will be hard, but just embrace it. Understand that life is going to suck asshole sometimes. If you do what is easy, your life will be hard but if you do what is hard your life will be easy. Those are the famous words from Les Brown.

Make supplements a bonus to your routine once you actually start creating a system in your life where you're being active each day whether it's working out at the gym a few days a week and maybe walking the dog on the weekend. Make sure you have those systems in your life and their consistent. Don't expect to take supplements and sit on your ass and eat like a dick head and expect to see results. Think about something that you're really good at. Were you just good out of nowhere? Or did you implement systems on a daily basis to get better and better at it? Did you go to school for 10 years or 15 years? When you were going to school did you have do homework and take test after test? After those years were you smarter? Do your homework. If that means writing down your data and seeing your progression, or taking a monthly photo to seeing your progression, whatever it may be that motivates you to accomplish your goals then do it.

If you're not drinking enough water on a daily basis then make that a goal and do it. Drink a lot. Wake up and drink water and tell yourself that you're detoxifying your body and you're getting healthier. That water is your fucking fat burner! Get your mind right! Don't tell yourself that you're fat. Compliment yourself and be happy with the little things that you get right. You are going to be the only person for a while that is going to believe in you. Make it a ritual every day to believe in you and never give up. As long as you never give up then you can never fail. Look at the greats for inspiration. Michael Jordan had one of his best games when he was deathly sick. I don't think it was deathly, but he felt like shit. The reason he did so good was because he was so freaking dedicated to being great at basketball. He listened to himself and he understood what needed to be done and he did day in and day out. He didn't care what others said because he knew that was just smoke and dust that didn't matter. All that mattered was that he progressed, worked hard and did what he knew he had to do. Those things that you feel deep down in your heart that God or the Universe is telling you to do.

I've taken a lot of natural supplements from creatine, to vitamins, to pre workouts, all the way to protein powders and yes they worked, but I guarantee you that the main reason they worked was because I was working hard and I had the correct belief systems. I laid a foundation down. I was working out 5 days a week or I was playing a sport, or I made healthy lifestyle choices and I did it consistently and I haven't stopped doing it. This is my lifestyle. I want to have 5 kids one day and I want to be a freak of nature when it comes to my body I want my kids to look up to me and get pumped up that their dad is healthy. I want to inspire people and let them know it's possible. You are possible. You are a phenomenal human being and it doesn't matter if you are fat or if you have an eating disorder or you have this disease that is keeping you from reaching your ultimate goal. If you feel like that is the only way to live, to be a victim then you will lose, but if you decide to make a personal decision, a strong affirmation to be great and to tell yourself you are in control and that you are making it happen as we speak because you are bad mother fucker and you are ready to kick ass! I am telling you, you will do great things.

I went from a little piece of shit in high school to some one that got really jacked and then losing it all because I was doing the exercise but I wasn't eating healthy. Then I had to go to the hospital for 20 days, got depressed and looked like shit but then it hit me I can't give up. I can't be a little baby. I need to get my life together. I need to do this for myself, but also for the people that love me and if no one loves you don't make that an excuse for why you can't get the body you want. Improve yourself and be active! Get the body you want! Get the life you want, be a power house that is unstoppable in life and not only are you getting the body you want but you're living a life full of balance. You don't stress over little things! You just crush life and you make shit happen!

If you want to take supplements, take supplements. It might help you get to your goal quicker, but remember there is no magic pill or magic button. You have to work, that is life. It sucks, but you have to work for everything that you want. You might have everything going wrong in your life right now, but that's mainly because you're asking for it and you know it because you are smart. You know you can't allow people to feel sorry for yourself because if you do that than those people will be talking behind your back wishing you would grow up, wishing you would stop being so negative, wishing you would better yourself. Don't allow yourself to be a victim of anything, anybody can do that, but if you play the victim and you don't forgive those people and events that have happened in your life then you will have a sad life because no one is going to care about you as much as you care about yourself. Start acting like a champion because you are already capable of being a champion.

Change your mindset. Create a game plan and be ready to work and see the hard work pay off because it will. If you do it consistently eventually it's going to work. That is how life works, nothing will be handed to you and if it is you will not respect it and you will lose it. If you take the money away from every billionaire they will get it back because they know how money works. They don't spend it, they invest it. Invest in yourself. Take today and invest in yourself do something nice to your body. Pick up a green smoothie, pick up a dumbbell, start running, challenge yourself, be great, you know you can do this, it is already in you! I believe in you.

Conclusion

Getting in shape isn't always easy. It can take a lot of time and it definitely requires you to put in a lot of effort. You will need to take care of your mind and body as well, but by putting all of these methods into effect you're going to feel better about yourself and you're actually going to feel better in general as well. That's because eating right and getting exercise is going to keep your entire body working properly and it's going to prolong your entire life (as well as helping you live a better life). There is no right diet. Groups of scientist have even done a study on diets and as long as you are adhering to some healthy lifestyle or if you want to call it a diet then you will see results. Figure out what works for your body. Not everyone wants to do paleo or ketogenic diet which in my opinion is a bullshit diet, but people see results with it. I just don't think it's healthy. What I am trying to get at is start today do something healthy for your body and be consistent.

By taking all this information into effect you're going to be prepared for even more and you're going to be ready to start your body transformation journey. So take some time to read through everything and start putting them into motion. By adding water, switching up your exercise plan and simply setting goals you're going to be well on your way to getting everything you've ever wanted. So start making goals. Start setting up your vision board and make it work for you. You're going to love everything that you get and it's all just the beginning.

We all have to go through crap in life but I am telling you if you want to have the dream body of your life and you do these things that I ask you to do. You will start to see results. Write down three things you want to accomplish today. Make one of them towards your health because right now you're dying. We're all dying and if we don't get that through our heads then we won't get to accomplish very much in life. But you still have a chance! Start being grateful for what you already have in your life and get more out of it! Life doesn't have to be hard, it can be very fun and you can achieve anything you want.

Dream big! You want to be a super model or a star football player in the NFL then do it. If you can visualize it in your head then it's possible. You might be thinking each and every day that your fat and unworthy and guess what your right. You are always right in some sense. You cannot expect someone to applaud you and tell you that you are great. You have to take that yourself. You have to be the one that says I'm going to make it. I am going to win. I am good looking. I feel great. I am amazing. I am unstoppable. I am accomplishing my dreams. I am happy. Those have to be your decisions. If you can't say it then no one will.

Join Our Facebook Groups

Make Life Your Beach is a mastermind group that I started with people that are goal oriented, crushing life and that have been a positive influence for me. We're always trying to grow Make Life Your Beach so you can always email us at makelifeyourbeachgroup@gmail.com to join our mastermind group but in the mean time you can check out our other Facebook groups for each section. We have 4 different sections that complete Make Life Your Beach. These 4 groups are free to join. Make Life Your Beach does have a yearly membership fee, but before we even get into that if you are interested just email us discussing why you believe you would be a great fit to the team and let us know what you are working on to better yourself and society.

Make Life Your Body Facebook group is used for keeping yourself and others accountable with their Health, Nutrition, Fitness and any other related goals to the body. You can post videos; you can write down your goals, you can share anything that has helped you. As long as it's related to making your health and fitness better.

Make Life Your Bank Facebook group is used for building your financial empire. You can share financial and career goals or how you were able to become financially free. Anything that is related to building your wealth and that you believe would help others become successful you may post in this group.

Make Life Your Babe Facebook group is used for building healthy relationships. Whether it's getting advice on marriage or having healthy relationships with family and friends. It can even be tips on finding the right person for you or the right people to surround yourself with. As long as you are posting information that is related to building relationships and finding love.

Make Life Your Book Facebook group is used for anything that makes you happy. Maybe it's a passion for music or art. You can use this platform to share your happiness. It could be tips on having a positive attitude or creating a great perspective towards life. It could be pictures of different places you traveled to or maybe you just bought your dream car and you can share it in this group. Or you can even make yourself accountable by posting a video and telling us what you plan on accomplishing with your life that is going to bring you happiness.

If You Enjoyed Reading This Book I Have Also Written Another Top Seller on Amazon! You Can Click the Picture of the Book Below and it will take You Directly to the Amazon Website for Download! I Hope You Enjoyed The Weight Loss Diet Guide as much as I Enjoyed Writing It!

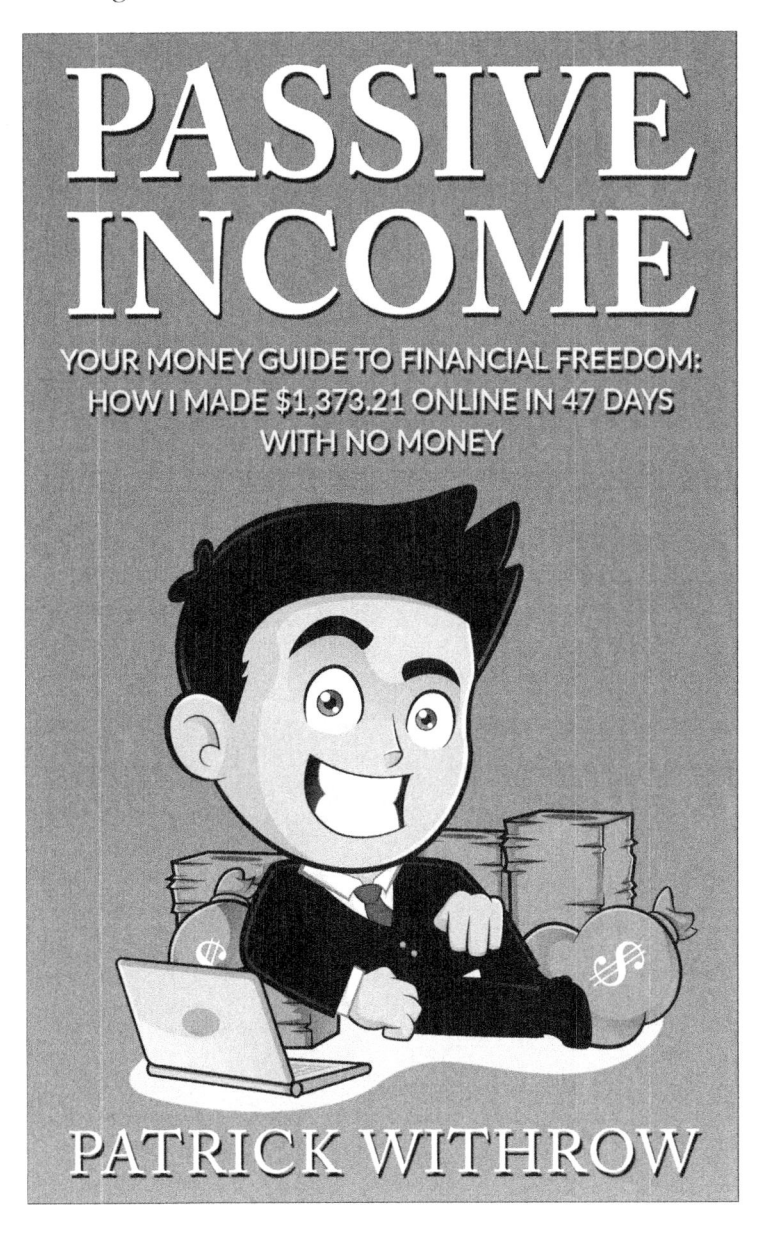

Printed in Great Britain
by Amazon